YOUR KNOWLEDGE HAS VALUE

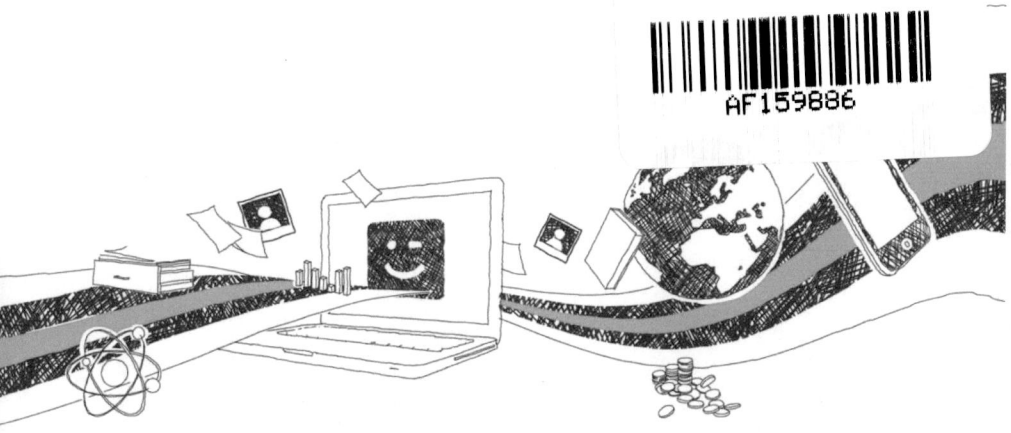

- We will publish your bachelor's and master's thesis, essays and papers

- Your own eBook and book - sold worldwide in all relevant shops

- Earn money with each sale

Upload your text at www.GRIN.com and publish for free

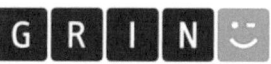

Bibliographic information published by the German National Library:

The German National Library lists this publication in the National Bibliography; detailed bibliographic data are available on the Internet at http://dnb.dnb.de .

This book is copyright material and must not be copied, reproduced, transferred, distributed, leased, licensed or publicly performed or used in any way except as specifically permitted in writing by the publishers, as allowed under the terms and conditions under which it was purchased or as strictly permitted by applicable copyright law. Any unauthorized distribution or use of this text may be a direct infringement of the author s and publisher s rights and those responsible may be liable in law accordingly.

Imprint:

Copyright © 2017 GRIN Verlag, Open Publishing GmbH
Print and binding: Books on Demand GmbH, Norderstedt Germany
ISBN: 9783668397811

This book at GRIN:

http://www.grin.com/en/e-book/353514/primary-care-provider-shortage

Pohl Ron

Primary Care Provider Shortage

An Evaluation of Three Policy Intervention Proposals

GRIN Publishing

GRIN - Your knowledge has value

Since its foundation in 1998, GRIN has specialized in publishing academic texts by students, college teachers and other academics as e-book and printed book. The website www.grin.com is an ideal platform for presenting term papers, final papers, scientific essays, dissertations and specialist books.

Visit us on the internet:

http://www.grin.com/

http://www.facebook.com/grincom

http://www.twitter.com/grin_com

Title: Primary Care Provider Shortage Proposal

Contents

Executive Summary 1
Organization Information 1
Background 2
Statement of Need 3
Proposed Plan 5
Plan 1: Altering the undergraduate medical education (UME) pathway in the two medical schools in the state 5
Plan 2: Increasing visa-waivers and improving loan-forgiveness and direct incentive programs 6
Plan 3: Increase residency funding 6
Project Evaluation 7
Conclusion 7
Sources cited 8

PRIMARY CARE PROVIDER SHORTAGE PROPOSAL

Executive Summary

We are proposing the following solutions to the challenge of primary healthcare provider shortages in rural Washington: that undergraduate medical education (UME) pathway in the two medical schools in the state be altered; visa-waivers, loan-forgiveness and direct incentive programs expanded; and residency funding be increased. These are workable with the right support and resources.

We understand that primary healthcare physician shortages will worsen more and more over the next decade if nothing is done now; and there is no doubt that communities have been feeling the impacts of shortages. Since none of the plans proposed here can work to reduce the expected decrease, the right combination of strategies will results in an increase in the number of primary healthcare physicians per population in rural Washington, which is the main aim of this proposal.

Organization Information

This proposal reflects the opinions of Neon Healthcare Research, a major research division of Neon Inc. We are a non-profit organization that aims at improving public health policies through the use of scientific research methods and solutions. We are focused on improving health and healthcare delivery in the United States and around the world. We have a broad research portfolio which ranges from newer challenges in the delivery of healthcare to emerging issues in non-communicable disease management and population health. Alongside this broad focus, we are particularly interested in a few key areas of health: organizing patient care, payment for health care, quality of care, health research tools, and healthy communities.

The recipient organization is the Washington State legislature who needs research and empirical support to make necessary policy changes in order to address the present shortage of primary care health care personnel in rural areas of the state.

Background

Primary healthcare has been the cornerstone on which strong healthcare systems have been built over the years as it ensures that communities experience positive health outcomes and health equity (Leiyu, 2012). There is presently a shift from disease-oriented etiologies to finding out what environmental, cultural, individual, and family factors are responsible for disease. This shift has led to a transition towards the provision of individual/family-oriented and community-focused healthcare services in a coordinated and sustainable manner so as to meet the health needs of the population. However, despite the understanding that primary health care is very vital to any healthcare system, many locations globally are experiencing imbalances between primary and secondary healthcare – including the United States. This has been referred to as primary healthcare provider shortage.

Primary healthcare provider shortage refers to the situation in which there is a reduction in the amount of local primary healthcare provider/physicians per capita below a particular threshold (Friedberg et al, 2016). According to the Health Resources and Services Administration (HRSA), primary care provider shortage areas are those locations in which the ratio of the primary care physician to the rest of the population is less than 1/3,500 (Friedberg et al, 2016). In the United States, the total number of primary healthcare physicians have been placed at 6,000 for a population of about 60 million people (Health Resources and Services Administration, 2015). Despite these glaring figures, the existence of primary healthcare physician shortages has not been completely accepted by the relevant stakeholders. A recent report from the Institute of Medicine showed that there was "no credible evidence" to support the claims that there were looming shortages in primary healthcare deliver (Pauly, Naylor, & Weiner, 2014).

It is understood that the fraction of primary care physicians who practice in the rural areas is very low compared to the urban centers. The presence of constant migration has negatively influenced the supply of skilled providers to these rural centers in which the rural primary care physicians are the older, and most probably, male, physicians who have been born in those locations (McGrail, 2015; Fordyce, Doescher, & Skillman, 2013). In Washington State, the total physician workforce was about 19,260 in strength as at 2014 (approximately 275 per 100,000 people), out of which 15,421 were into direct patient care (at 220/100,000 population) (Friedberg et al, 2016). From figures obtained at the end of 2015, 154 primary healthcare shortage areas were discovered within which a population of about 1,291,074 lived. These areas needed up to 229 additional primary healthcare physicians to meet the minimum requirements, even though this shortage has been predicted to increase to about 1695 physicians needed by 2030 in rural Washington.

The present bulk of primary healthcare physicians in Washington State are fed mainly by a pipeline of graduates from the University Of Washington School Of Medicine, and the Pacific Northwest University of Health Sciences (PNWU). The former, being an allopathic medical school produces about 200 medical graduates per year, focusing on general medical practice, while the latter is an osteopathic medical school which graduates about 140 students per year (Skillman & Stover, 2014; Greer et al, 2016).

In 2014, the state of Washington had about 1900 residents who vied for the Accreditation Council for Graduate Medical Education (ACGME)-sponsored training programs during which these residents experience rural rotations and contribute to the rural primary healthcare physician workforce (Friedberg et al, 2016). This is equivalent to about 27 physicians per 100,000 population, lower than the general state median of 27.4 resident trainees per 100,000 population. According to Friedberg et al (2016), the University of Washington's Family Medicine Residency Network and its allied rural medicine training programs have been able to retain residents in rural medical practice after the completion of training. However, these programs have experienced significant funding and other logistical challenges (Lesko, Fitch, & Pauwels, 2011).

In addition to the state-produced graduates of medicine, a survey of medical practitioners who received J-1 visa waivers between 1993 and 2003 showed that 84 percent of these people stayed longer than the required 3- to 5-year commitment with employers, 57 percent stayed back in Washington to continue their practice, and 91 percent practiced in urban areas (Kahn, Hagopian & Johnson, 2010).

Statement of Need

In this section, present the results of your research into the issue based on the perspective/organization(s) you have selected. Determine the scope of your focus, for example a geographic area, economic level, and/or ethnic group. Discuss problems faced in addressing the identified needs and any previous actions taken to deal with this need. Identify potential opportunities for implementing change.

As the demand for healthcare services in the rural areas increase, and the shortages of primary healthcare physicians worsens, patients and the rest of the Washington rural communities will bear the full brunt. As stated previously. The present primary healthcare physician workforce is made up of by about 19,000 doctors, majority of which are into general patient care.

When populations are blessed with an increased supply of primary healthcare providers, research has shown that there will be improved health outcomes in the form of reduced mortality, optimal birth weights, longer life expectancies, and improved self-related health (Starfield, Shi & Macinko, 2005; Friedberg, Hussey, & Schneider, 2010). In addition, greater supply has been associated with increased focus on preventive health care (earlier detection of cancers), and a reduction in health inequalities related to income disparities (Chang, O'Malley, & Goodman, 2016).

Shortage of primary healthcare providers have been associated with worse healthcare access, more hospital admissions and requirement of secondary care, and increased emergency room visits (Pathman, Ricketts, & Konrad, 2006; Liu, 2007; Chang, O'Malley, & Goodman, 2016).

It is important to note that some policy interventions have been made recently to address primary healthcare provider shortage in rural Washington State. This includes the changing of the law that gives the University of Washington the monopoly of operating a medical school in the state, and also funding the start-up of a new medical school at Washington State University (WSU). The new school which has received preliminary accreditation is expected to have its first medical class matriculate in 2017. Also, there has been an increase in the available funding budget aimed at supporting Washington's primary health care graduate medical education program so as to allows for the opening of additional residency slots. In addition, there has been creation of medical home models which assist in enhancing access to primary healthcare.

In other states that have used some of these policy interventions, significant improvements have been recorded as regards the amelioration of primary care physician shortages. Many states in the US have recently added new medical schools or expanded existing ones, leading to an increase in medical student enrolment (Erikson, Whatley, & Hampton, 2015). Expansion of residency programs has led to an increase in the number of residency trainees, and evidences have shown that these graduates are more likely to practice in underserved rural settings (Ku et al, 2015). Findings are ambiguous as regard the long-term benefits of National Health Service Corps scholarships and other direct financial incentive programs in relation to their contribution to improving primary care workforce in rural areas. However, some studies have found that physicians who enjoy these benefits are more likely than their peers to settle in rural primary care practice (Porterfield et al, 2003; Pathman, Konrad, & Ricketts, 1992).

Proposed Plan

It is clear that the challenge of ameliorating the shortage of primary care physician is immense, but the proposed plan is simple. The goal is to improve primary health care delivery in Washington's rural communities; while the specific objectives are:

- To encourage and increase the training of physicians who can deliver primary health care
- To stimulate interest in rural family medicine practice in the state

Plan 1: Altering the undergraduate medical education (UME) pathway in the two medical schools in the state

The aim of this plan is to encourage and increase the amount of students that decide to go for a profession in family medicine. The specifics are to create about 20 – 30 spots each out of the total 200 and 140 spots in the University Of Washington School Of Medicine and the Pacific Northwest University of Health Sciences respectively. This will help generate an additional 40 to 60 additional PGY-1 interns in family medicine every year. Then benefit of this program is to have not more than 6 years of medical education in total, and a facilitated entry into family medicine residency.

In addition to the above, this plan alleviates many of the concerns associated with traditional medical education in the United States such as financial stress and college debt. This program is less expensive than the usual 4-year medical program during which many family medicine residents would have accumulated up to $150,000 in debts by the time they are completing their program. Also, it gives the added advantage of increased connectivity as the usual transition from undergraduate medical education to residency is not smooth for the majority of students presently. However, this plan eases the transition. Again, it affords the opportunity for improved longitudinal tracking for the students based on their clinical skills, performance evaluations, and interaction with patients.

Critics of this accelerated pathway claim that three-years of undergraduate medical education is not enough, and this is difficult to disclaim as there is presently limited data to prove otherwise. However, this accelerated program offers the option of exiting if the student feels the program is too intense or wants a change in specialty. It also raises the concern of choice as students who come in through this pathway must be committed to family medicine. However, since there is a much needed role for these students to fill after graduation, there is less worry about them finding a job when they finally finish.

Plan 2: Increasing visa-waivers and improving loan-forgiveness and direct incentive programs

It is understood that the state of Washington has instituted loan-forgiveness programs such as the state-funded Health Professional Loan Repayment Program, even though the budget was cut down drastically from $8.7 million to about $1 million in 2011 (Friedberg et al, 2016). This was later increased in 2015 back to $9.6 million (Washington State Medical Association, 2015). However, much more can be done. Asides this, many community health centers in rural communities face difficulties in getting primary care physicians, and their hope rests only on physicians in these loan-repayment programs, on J-1 visa waivers, or on the National Health Service Corps (NHSC) scholarships. It is believed that doing more to increase these incentives will further boost the number of primary care physicians in rural locations in the state.

Plan 3: Increase residency funding

The present slots available per year in family medicine residency are limited mostly by the funds available at that time. In order to support the primary healthcare physician workforce pipeline earlier described, additional funding will do a lot of good in supporting Washington's graduate medical program, and opening more slots for residency in the University of Washington. Having more slots will also encourage students graduating from the newly proposed medical school to decide to go for a residency in family medicine.

Workability: To achieve these two plans, it is essential to collaborate with necessary stakeholders in the Washington State Medical Association, the Washington State Health Care Authority, the state legislature's Liaison Committee on Medical Education, the authorities of the two medical schools in the state, and other relevant stakeholders. The essence of this collaboration will be to propose these plans to them, present evidences that support their feasibility, and discuss how to implement these programs within the limits of available resources. This can be achieved within a timeline of six to nine months if all stakeholders are willing to collaborate and work on these plans.

The resources required will include funds budgeted and released by the state legislature through the relevant coordinating agencies, personnel who will direct specific aspects of these plans,

Project Evaluation

It is understood that this is a complex challenge, even though the proposed solutions appear simple. It becomes necessary to evaluate these solutions as soon as implementation begins to ensure that they follow the plan and they also help to achieve the intended objectives. In evaluating this plan, the following targets will be measured to assess the progress being made:

1. The number of slots available for family medicine residency per year.
2. The number of students who choose a family medicine career every year.

Conclusion

Primary healthcare physician shortages will worsen more and more over the next decade if nothing is done now. None of the plans proposed here can work to reduce the expected decrease, but this combination of strategies will results in an increase in the number of primary healthcare physicians per population in rural Washington, which is the main aim of this proposal.

Sources cited

Chang, C., O'Malley, J., & Goodman, D. C. Association between temporal changes in primary care workforce and patient outcomes. *Health Services Research*, June 3, 2016.

Erikson, C., Whatley, M., & Hampton, S. (2015). *Results of the 2014 medical school enrollment survey*, Washington, D.C.: Association of American Medical Colleges, Center for Workforce Studies. Retrieved from: https://members.aamc.org/eweb/upload/Results%20of%20the%202014%20Medical%20School%20Enrollment%20Survey.pdf

Fordyce, M. A., Doescher, M. P., & Skillman, S. M. (2013). *The aging of the rural primary care physician workforce: will some locations be more affected than others?* Seattle, Wash.: University of Washington, School of Medicine. Retrieved from: http://depts.washington.edu/uwrhrc/uploads/RHRC_FR127_Fordyce.pdf

Friedberg, M. W., Hussey, P. S., & Schneider, E. C. (2010). Primary care: a critical review of the evidence on quality and costs of health care. *Health Affairs*, 29(5), 766–772.

Friedberg, M. W., Martsolf, G. R., White, C., Auerbach, D. I., Kandrack, R., Reid, R. O., Butcher, E., Yu, H., Hollands, S., & Nie, X. (2016). *Evaluation of policy options for increasing the availability of primary care services in rural Washington State*. California: RAND Corporation.

Greer, T., Kost, A., Evans, D. V., Norris, T, Erickson, J., McCarthy, J., & Allen, S. (2016). The WWAMI targeted rural underserved track (TRUST) program: an innovative response to rural physician workforce shortages. *Academic Medicine*, 91(1), 65–69.

Health Resources and Services Administration. (2015). *Data warehouse, preformatted reports: MUA/P by state and county*. Retrieved from: http://datawarehouse.hrsa.gov/tools/hdwreports/Filters.aspx?id=52

Kahn, T. R., Hagopian, A., & Johnson, K. (2010). Retention of J-1 visa waiver program physicians in Washington State's health professional shortage areas. *Academic Medicine*, 85(4), 614–621.

Ku, L., Mullan, F., Serrano, C., Barber, Z., & Shin, P. (2015). *Teaching health centers: a promising approach for building primary care workforce for the 21st century*. Geiger

Gibson Program in Community Health Policy and RCHN Community Health Foundation Research Collaborative, Policy Research Brief 40. Retrieved from: http://www.rchnfoundation.org/?p=4651

Leiyu, S. (2012). The impact of primary care: A focused review. *Scientifica*, 2012(432892), 1-22.

Lesko, S., Fitch, W., & Pauwels, J. (2011). Ten-year trends in the financing of family medicine training programs: considerations for planning and policy. *Family Medicine*, 43(8), 543–550.

Liu, J. (2007). Health professional shortage and health status and health care access. *Journal of Health Care for the Poor and Underserved*, 18(3), 590–598.

McGrail, M. (2015). *Rurality and community amenity: how they relate to rural primary care supply and workforce retention*, Australian Primary Health Care Research Institute and Robert Graham Center Visiting Fellowship, 2014 report. Retrieved from: http://aphcri.anu.edu.au/files/McGrail_RGCFull%20report.pdf

Pathman, D. E., Konrad, T. R., & Ricketts III, T. C. (1992). The comparative retention of national health service corps and other rural physicians: results of a 9-year follow-up study. *JAMA*, 268(12), 1552–1558.

Pathman, D. E., Ricketts, T. C., & Konrad, T. R. How adults' access to outpatient physician services relates to the local supply of primary care physicians in the rural southeast. *Health Services Research*, 41(1), 79–102.

Pauly, M. V., Naylor, M., & Weiner, J. (2014). *Primary care shortages: it's more than just a head count*. Robert Wood Johnson Foundation

Porterfield, D. S., Konrad, T. R., Porter, C. Q., Leysieffer, K., Martinez, R. M., Niska, R., Wells, B., & Potter, F. (2003). Caring for the underserved: current practice of alumni of the national health service corps. *Journal of Health Care for the Poor and Underserved*, 14(2), 256–271.

Skillman, S. M., & Stover, B. (2014). *Washington State's physician workforce in 2014*. Seattle, Wash.: WWAMI Center for Health Workforce Studies, University of Washington.

Retrieved from: http://depts.washington.edu/uwrhrc/uploads/CHWS_WA_Phys_Workforce_2014.pdf

Starfield, B., Shi, L., & Macinko, J. (2005). Contribution of primary care to health systems and health. *Milbank Quarterly*, 83(3), 457–502.

Washington State Medical Association. (2015). *Legislative session wrap-up*. Retrieved from: http://www.wsma.org/doc_library/GovernmentAffairs/LegislativeAdvocacy/2015_WSMA_LegWrapUp.pdf

YOUR KNOWLEDGE HAS VALUE

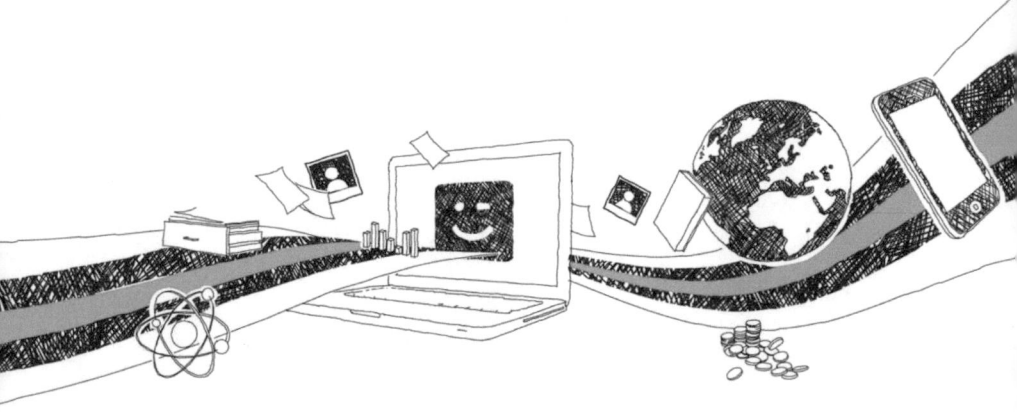

- We will publish your bachelor's and master's thesis, essays and papers

- Your own eBook and book - sold worldwide in all relevant shops

- Earn money with each sale

Upload your text at www.GRIN.com
and publish for free

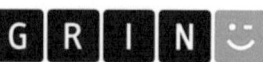